AF484666

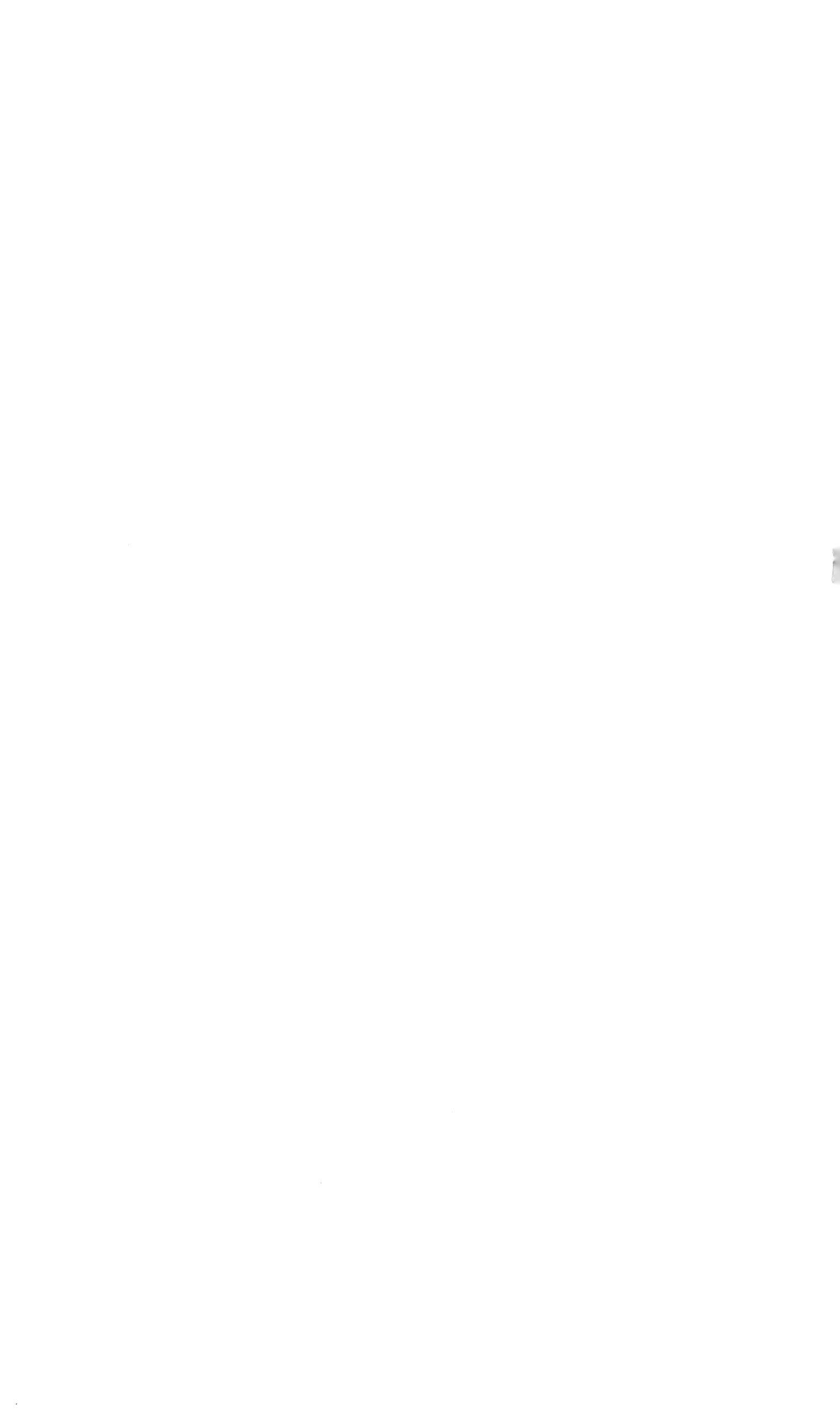

Alcoholics Anonymous and its Spiritual Approach

Our Incorrect Core Premises Are Invisible and Thus Spiritual?

Loran Joly

Foreword

This book is much more of an outline of major ideas on alcoholism and its "treatment", than it is a polished work.

It is a way of my getting started on what I have spent a whole lifetime around....

But am now at the point where life is so very challenging in its own ways at the age of sixty-three....

And so, isn't a Bird in the Hand worth a whole Sky-Full of Birds that may never come flying by?

For this is just the beginning, actually, of a whole "ton" of works in this and other areas, as I will later explain more.

And too, it is a way for me to open a dialog with others in this area, by which we can discuss the ideas I bring up here.

Chapter 1

This book is Imperfect!

This book is a conversation and certainly not polished, in certain ways....

However, I do believe that the logic behind the ideas in this short book are likely quite sound.

Furthermore, let us not be confused by its few number of pages or lack of considerable price-point?

So, to begin with,

I believe that the beginning of a Journey starts with the first step.

And what more essential step than to come to believe that we are not perfect?

In terms of our core premises, that is?

For we all know that we are not perfect at our job tasks or knowledge about the ways things work around us.

But what about when it comes to our premises?

* * *

It appears to this author, that a massive change happens, if and when we human beings come to see that we were incorrect in one or more of our core premises.

And where alcohol overuse is concerned - "alcoholism" - that this involves making no real progress with this burden **until one comes to change one or more core premises -** call it the changing of one or two kingpin ***"Stinking Thinking Premises"***, if you will.

* * *

Namely, ***the change to a core belief that we <u>cannot</u> alter the Laws of the Universe, in order to make our lives happier.***

* * *

And why would we think we could alter the Laws of the Universe?

Perhaps this happens if we think of ourselves as able to "Pull a Rabbit Out of a Hat", or follow the adage of "Where There's a Will, There's a Way": without regard to either the necessary Resources, and necessary Freedom from anything Constraining: two key concepts in the mathematical field of

Operations Research ("resources and constraints" being addressed constantly, in goal-setting, as this author found out when he took a graduate level mathematics class in Operations Research, a few years after West Point.)

Chapter 2

We Have Leaped Ahead If And When...

Hence it is the author's view that the key phrase in Alcoholics Anonymous - AA - of "Turn your life over to a Higher Power" - is everything, actually, of **turning *Away From Oneself* as that *Higher Power*** - in the sense of FORMERLY **having thought of ourselves as <u>*A Power Capable of Breaking the Laws of the Universe.*</u>**

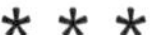

In other words, it is coming to realize that we are not Magicians; we are not able to make something happen out of thin air. That we cannot Magically make things happen or keep from happening.

Chapter 3

If We Think We Are Magicians...

To put it another way, the idea of a Higher Power being simply the dawn of seeing that ***to turn to a Higher Power could be said to turn to The Power of Reality,*** as opposed to **The Power of Wishful Thinking** - the Power of a Magician that can't actually do any Magic Tricks....

Or, as Einstein said of his God, his Higher Power:
"God Does Not Play Dice With the Universe";
Everything said to follow Laws, call these Laws of the Universe, or the Laws of God or Gods, or Laws of a Higher Power.

Which surely is not simply a more Effective Power than Wishful Thinking, or Magical Thinking, if you will, but the ONLY ACTUAL way of seeing things sanely - hence Higher in this sense!

On the other hand, to believe we *have* the Power to Transcend the Laws of the Universe, could be said to be a Lower Power - because it is quite impotent. It doesn't work, in other words.

* * *

Put another way, it is neither a Higher Power, nor even a Lower Power, but a NONSENSICAL Power - a Power that will doom us to a life of misery, because it lacks any STRENGTH.

Chapter 4

Let Go and Let God?

So, perhaps the phrase "Let Go and Let God", too, could be said to mean,

"Let Go of thinking we are Magicians with the name of

"I Can Have Anything I Desire, and Immediately, Too",

and turning instead, to the core idea - core belief - as put forth in the phrase, "Let God" - let the Laws of the Universe, even - be what makes things happen or not happen....

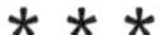

* * *

Or, put another way, this example:

a shift from thinking that we can make a wonderful turkey dinner, by simply snapping our fingers?

In favor of coming to accept that the Laws of the Universe dictate that we actually put a turkey in the oven, set the temperature properly, and roast it for a certain period of time?

We thus "Let Go" of the desire to make a Turkey Dinner happen by wishful thinking, and "turn" to a "Higher Power" to make the dinner - or NOT - in ACCORDANCE to The Laws of the Universe:

* * *

And this Higher Power, then, arguably is the Laws of Physics.

Put another way, "If you put in this substance, and subject it to xyz conditions and what not, the outcome is Guaranteed - by the Laws of the Universe.

* * *

Because OUTCOMES to not follow WHIMSY - or RANDOMNESS - but instead, they follow Procedures? Rules? Protocol, if you will?

And if we expect things to happen any differently, isn't that quite a way to not have that nice dinner?

Put another way, "do nothing, get nothing",

"No turkey IN the oven, and there WON'T any Turkey coming OUT of the oven and on to the table!"

Chapter 5

The Confusing Issue of Saying That Some Things Are in Our Control?

Now, if we say, though, "Turn your life over to a Higher Power" - or acknowledge that anything and everything that happens is in accord with the Laws of the Universe, then how can it also be said, then, that some things are "In our Control", while other things are "NOT in our Control", as per the Serenity Prayer?

> *"God, grant me the serenity to accept the things I cannot change, Courage to change the things I can,*
> *And wisdom to know the difference."*
> — Reinhold Niebuhr

* * *

Well, my own view on this phrase that that there are SOME things we CAN "***Change***", means simply this:

· · ·

That there is a great _likelihood_ that something positive WILL come about - the reducing of a certain Pain Point, or a certain Painful Situation - IF we can acquire the necessary RESOURCES, before we die.

* * *

As an example, it is surely likely, that if our car runs out of gas as we are driving, that we _will_ be <u>able</u> to get more gas for it, or get a tow truck, before we die.

And so, we call such a thing something that "we <u>CAN</u> CHANGE": because the <u>SITUATION</u> is <u>LIKELY</u> to CHANGE - SOMEHOW.

* * *

But on the OTHER hand, if we wish the car to CHANGE into a SPACESHIP, or PUT IT on our BACKS and WALK HOME with this car, without needing to call for assistance or get gas in some way, then THIS DESIRE to ALTER the LAWS of the UNIVERSE, are NOT "IN" our "CON-TROL", is it?

Chapter 6

But Then What Can Be Changed?

So, those things that Niebuhr said we can CHANGE, are perhaps, precisely those things that we are LIKELY to SOMEDAY get the RESOURCES for, or see certain CONSTRAINTS CHANGE, in our LIFETIME.

And whether we can or cannot get these RESOURCES, is again, arguably a matter precisely of the Laws of the Universe....

* * *

BUT, and yes, BUT, it being far more LIKELY, that we tend to SEE the Laws of the Universe PLAY in our DESIRED FAVOR, EVENTUALLY, in CERTAIN areas, like GETTING GAS for our car, ***rather than the UNLIKELY scenario, that this car TURN INTO a SPACESHIP.***

. . .

And so, it seems to this author that we use, as verbal SHORTHAND, that it is "IN our CONTROL" to GET GASOLINE, in that it is thus FAR MORE LIKELY that a GOOD SAMARITAN will come along and GIVE us some gas, or we can alternatively CALL someone for ASSISTANCE with GETTING gas.

* * *

On the other hand, it being said, to **NOT be "in our CONTROL", we say, to TURN a SODA or bottle of WATER into GAS, EVER.**

* * *

Again, it being LIKELY we WILL get GAS, SOMEHOW - this then termed "GETTING GAS, to be something "IN our 'CONTROL'",

because it is LIKELY we WILL, ONEDAY, GET some gas; but UTTERLY UN-likely that we will EVER be ABLE to TURN AIR or WATER into GAS: this MAGIC, thus, said, in "verbal shorthand", to NOT "Be in our 'Control'".

Chapter 7

The Concept of Forgiveness and the AA Way...

Now, if a Core Principle of AA is to have a Higher Power view, then how does this tie in to "Forgiveness"?

* * *

The author sees Forgiveness as simply the coming to conclude that a situation could not have been ANY DIFFERENT than it WAS or IS - by way of the Laws of the Universe.

Or, thus, that if we felt pain in connection with encounters with someone else, that it was _inevitable_, both in terms of what went into making the other person, as well as what has made us interpret any and all experiences in a way that may well amplify the pain we feel.

And so, to "forgive" someone, is likely to be to say,

"The other person could not have been any other than who they were," first of all.

.   .   ,

And secondly, too, that we somehow say, even, "I forgive MYSELF, too, in the sense of seeing what WENT INTO my NOT being able to INTERPRET the pain in a way that MADE it LESS INTENSE, by far."

* * *

And the OUTCOME to such?

An end to the pain of a lot of ANGER, and too, constantly saying, "you could have done other than you did" - or, "you could have BEEN Other than you WERE - IF ONLY you had 'TRIED HARDER'" - "If only "YOU had BEEN ABLE to BEAT the LAWS of the UNIVERSE and BE or DO DIFFERENTLY than you DID!"

"IF ONLY you HAD been ABLE to BE a MAGICIAN and DO MAGIC TRICKS for yourself and me, too".

* * *

So, the final upshot being, a ceasing of "blame," in the sense of "I 'BLAME' you for NOT BEING a MAGICIAN"; and one also, of CEASING to SHAME ONESELF, in that one CEASES to continue to say, "I, TOO, COULD have BEEN a MAGICIAN, and done or been other than what The Laws of the Universe dictated."

And then, as the phrase goes, we stop "beating ourselves up" for what we WEREN'T WERE, or thus, "Didn't DO'", on ACCOUNT of our NOT BEING a MAGICIAN that supposedly CAN *OVERCOME* - *can FLOUT* - the LAWS of the UNIVERSE - the LAWS of CAUSE and EFFECT, thus.

This, then, putting into proper perspective, our otherwise unrealistic expectations of ourselves and others, and the associated shame and guilt issues and blame issues, so to speak.

Chapter 8

The Word Spiritual is Nothing Hokey?

So, to recap, it seems likely that the REORIENTATION to a view that ALL is GOVERNED by LAWS of CAUSE and EFFECT, or RECIPES, if you will, is in stark CONTRAST to the views so often found on a more COMFORTABLE plain - and for THIS reason, likely, it is said, that to come to SEE Life as a RECIPE, vs WISHFUL THINKING, is a "SPIRITUAL" way of Seeing Things, because it is a PHILOSOPHICAL way of interpreting our Pains - *a way based upon LOGIC - rather than ILLOGIC, if you will.*

* * *

And isn't the SEEING things - including the Pains we experience - through the INTANGIBLE of a LOGICAL CONCEPT - the very ESSENCE of something INTANGIBLE, yet still *THERE*?

* * *

Put another way, that LOGIC - and the PREMISES that reasoning is to take place by - are NOT VISIBLE to the eye, like a hamburger, or car, or house - yet, these LAWS of HOW THINGS WORK, are STILL THERE, hence, are called, in VERBAL SHORTHAND, the "Things" which are <u>SPIRI-TUAL</u> Objects, vs those things that are MORE EASY to SEE, and which, too, MOST people around us, ALSO AGREE are THERE?

And so, our CORE PREMISES being less SEE-ABLE, because LESS AGREED upon, we refer to as "SPIRITUAL" objects?

Chapter 9

We Can Have More of Life...

It is said,
"You can't have your cake and eat it too."
But perhaps we can say,
We can have a *better* way of life, if...?

* * *

For, the Way of Life that says, "<u>Anything</u> is possible," is comforting on an immediate level.

And yet, to not see that we are governed by Laws of the Universe, is to find ourselves inevitably setting goals for ourselves and others, that are not possibly able to come to be, at times.

Isn't it thus better that we have a limited view of what is possible - than to have goals that keep getting frustrated, when it comes to ourselves - and having unrealistic expectations for others, too, which also end up causing us "frustrated outcomes," and thus, again, anger?

And isn't anger arguably one of the biggest reasons to be unhappy, along with fear?

Chapter 10

There Surely is Always Hope - of Straightening Out Our Incorrect Premises

Our greatest hope, when greatly challenged?

Perhaps, to realize that most everything in life is neither Simple, nor Utterly Complex, on the other hand.

* * *

And secondly, that we likely suffer greatly until we learn certain key lessons - in particular, those lessons that we could call Core Lessons - about Reality as it is, not as we Wish it Were....

And until then, we keep returning the the Classes in Life, until we gain sufficient mastery?

. . .

And maybe this is what is happening when a person experiences relief through certain core beliefs in Alcoholics Anonymous?

21

To Contact the Author...

The author can be reached at message@goldpogo.com

Epilogue

The author has many credentials, including the Credential of Not Having a Ph.D. or MD degree. And the No College Degrees Credential - if one isn't referring to West Point as a College....

Noting, that he has studied more Electrical Engineering and Mathematics than one can shake a stick at.

And has applied the thinking skills from these areas to the areas of psychology - "people"; and to religion; and sociology; and much more.

And too, he has spent 150 sessions in psychoanalysis with two medical doctors, when he was in his twenties, including one hundred of such in San Diego, during the period of 1987-1990.

. . .

He also found his four years spent at West Point, invaluable, where he had sought to become a medical doctor.... But found it rather a bit much, and his grades slipped and had to reorient his life.

Indeed, his physical strength was never a great plus point, and so, West Point sought to beef him up by assigning him the sport of weightlifting with the West Point football team, his first Spring, there, and by eating with the football team members, too, for a period of time, where they and he received double rations of food....

Additionally, a Special Forces officer, who had earlier played on a professional baseball team, helped him mentally toughen up by requiring that he be a referee in intramural soccer one year, and deal with having to make split second decisions on the fields as a "ref", along with any "Ah, Ref"....

* * *

He later experienced many more things in his life, but credits the most to what he has learned from both observation and logic, as well as the Gift-Center of Pain.

As well as his parents and grandparents....

* * *

Other non-academic credentials include having overcome a whole host of physical ailments brought on, often, from the stressors of life, and incorrect premises and words to deal with these.

For, as his "ideas" improved, so too did his health.

More on this later....

There is of course much more to it all, including his immigrant upbringing, and time in inner city Detroit as a Kindergartner, and the influence of a lot of time on a farm, and in nature....

Again, more to follow....